Hairloss Solution

Natural Guide on how to prevent, control, treat hair loss, grey hair, dandruff, baldness, ringworm, folliculitis, psoriasis, alopecia, thinning hair (restore your hairline)

Barbara S. Johnson

Table of Contents

HAIRLOSS SOLUTION 1

INTRODUCTION 4

CHAPTER 1 5

    UNDERSTANDING HAIR LOSS 5

    CAUSES OF CURLY HAIR LOSS 8

    HOW DO DOCTORS CLASSIFY HAIR LOSS? 18

CHAPTER 2 21

    19 HERBAL TREATMENTS FOR HAIR REGROWTH 21

    POSSIBLE SIDE EFFECTS AND RISKS 30

CHAPTER 3 34

    30 NATURAL HERBS FOR HAIR REGROWTH AND THICKNESS 34

    16 WONDER HERBS THAT PREVENT HAIR LOSS 59

    12 WONDERFUL VEGETABLES FOR HAIR REGROWTH 84

    VEGETABLES FOR HAIR REGROWTH: 86

ACKNOWLEDGEMENTS 92

Copyright © 2022 by Barbara S. Johnson

All rights reserved. No part of this publication may be reproduced, distributed, or transmitted in any form or by any means, including photocopying, recording, or other electronic or mechanical methods, without the prior written permission of the publisher, except in the case of brief quotations embodied in critical reviews and certain other non-commercial uses permitted by copyright law.

Introduction

Hair grows everywhere on the human being pores and skin except on the hands of our hands and the bottoms of our ft, but many hairs are so fine they're practically invisible. Hair comprises of a proteins called keratin that is stated in hair roots in the external layer of epidermis. As follicles produce new curly hair cells, old cellular material are being forced out through the top of skin at the pace around six ins a 12 months. The hair you can see is truly a string of lifeless keratin cells. The common adult mind has about 100,000 to 150,000 hairs and manages to lose up to 100 of these each day; finding a few stray hairs on your hairbrush is definitely not cause for security alarm.

At anybody time, about 90% of the locks on someone's scalp keeps growing. Each follicle has its life cycle that may be affected by age group, disease, and a multitude of other factors.

Chapter 1

Understanding Hair Loss

Hair grows everywhere on the human being pores and skin except on the hands of our hands and the bottoms of our ft, but many hairs are so fine they're practically invisible. Hair comprises of a proteins called keratin that is stated in hair roots in the external layer of epidermis. As follicles produce new curly hair cells, old cellular material are being forced out through the top of skin at the pace around six ins a 12 months. The hair you can see is truly a string of lifeless keratin cells. The common adult mind has about 100,000 to 150,000 hairs and manages to lose up to 100 of these each day; finding a few stray hairs on your hairbrush is definitely not cause for security alarm.

At anybody time, about 90% of the locks on someone's scalp keeps growing. Each follicle has its life cycle that may be affected by age group, disease, and a multitude of other factors. This life routine is split into three stages:

- Anagen -- dynamic hair regrowth that is maintained between two to 6 years

- Catagen -- transitional hair regrowth that lasts 2-3 weeks

- Telogen -- resting stage that is maintained about 2-3 months; by the end of the relaxing phase the curly hair is shed and a fresh curly hair replaces it and the growing routine starts again.

As people age, their rate of hair growth slows.

There are various kinds of baldness, also known as alopecia:

- Involutional alopecia is an all natural condition where the hair steadily thins with age. More hair roots go in to the relaxing phase, and the rest of the hairs become shorter and fewer in quantity.

- Androgenic alopecia is a hereditary condition that make a difference men and women. Men with this problem, called male design baldness, can start suffering hair loss as soon as their teenagers or early 20s. It's seen as a receding hairline and progressive disappearance of locks from the crown and frontal head. Women with this problem, called female design hair loss, don't experience apparent loss until their 40s or later. Women experience an over-all loss over the whole scalp, with extensive hair loss at the crown.

- Alopeciareata often begins suddenly and causes patchy hair loss in children and adults. This problem may lead to complete hair loss (alopecia totalis). However in about 90% of individuals with the problem, the hair earnings within a couple of years.

- Alopecia universalis causes all body curly hair to fallout, like the eyebrows, eyelashes, and pubic locks.

- Trichotillomania , seen most regularly in children, is a psychological disorder when a person pulls out one's own curly hair.

- Telogen effluvium is short-term hair loss on the scalp occurring because of changes in the development cycle of locks. A lot of hairs enter the relaxing phase at exactly the same time, causing curly hair shedding and following loss.

- Scarring alopecias lead to permanent lack of locks. Inflammatory pores and skin conditions (cellulitis, folliculitis, acne), and other epidermis disorders (such as some types of lupus and lichen planus) often lead to marks that destroy the power of the curly hair to regenerate. Hot combs and locks too firmly woven and drawn can also lead to permanent hair loss.

Causes of curly hair loss

Possible factors behind hair loss include:

1. Androgenetic alopecia

Androgenetic alopecia is another term for female or male

pattern baldness. It really is an extremely common reason behind hair loss.

Both male and female pattern baldness is genetic. Men have a tendency to lose locks from the temples and crown of the top. In females, curly hair usually becomes leaner all around the head.

Androgenetic alopecia is much more likely to occur as a person ages but can begin at any point after puberty. Many females who experience androgenetic alopecia develop it after going right through the menopause. Which means that bodily hormones may have something regarding it.

You'll be able to regard this condition with minoxidil, a medication for hair regrowth.

2. Pregnancy

Some women may experience excessive hair loss shortly after having a baby. This is credited to a reduction in estrogen quantity. This sort of hair loss is a short-term condition and usually resolves within a yr or sooner.

To greatly help hair go back to its normal condition, try:

- using a volumizing shampoo and conditioner

- using products created for fine hair

- staying away from intensive conditioners or conditioning shampoos as these can be overweight for fine hair

- applying conditioner to the ends of the hair, as opposed to the head, to avoid weighing hair down

3. Telogen effluvium

Telogen effluvium is a disorder where the locks remains in the telogen (natural shedding) stage of the development routine. This causes more curly hair to fallout, sometimes in handfuls.

Telogen effluvium is generally a short-term condition that resolves as time passes. It is recommended to see a medical expert to discover the cause.

Some possible causes include:

- severe stress.

- Surgery.

- Childbirth.

- fast weight loss.

- thyroid problems.

- certain medications

A doctor should treat any underlying factors behind telogen effluvium.

If a health care provider suspects that specific medications are leading to hair loss, they could change them.

4. Anagen effluvium

Anagen effluvium causes giant amounts of locks to fallout rapidly through the anagen (development) stage of the curly hair cycle.

The condition could cause hair to fallout from the top, as well as from other areas of your body, including eyebrows and eyelashes.

Factors behind anagen effluvium include:

- chemotherapy.

- Radiation.

- fungal infections.

- autoimmune disease

Treatment because of this condition depends upon the reason but range from a topical solution of minoxidil.

If one has anagen effluvium consequently of undergoing chemotherapy, cooling the head during the process may help. Locks will most likely grow back again 3-6 weeks after preventing chemotherapy.

5. Alopeciareata

Alopeciareata can be an autoimmune condition that triggers hair to fallout suddenly. The disease fighting capability attacks hair roots, and also other healthy areas of the body.

Curly hair from the head, as well as eyebrows and eyelashes, may fallout in small chunks.

If one has this condition, they ought to see a medical expert. A health care provider may prescribe medication to help the locks grow back.

6. Traction alopecia

Grip alopecia is hair loss thanks to pulling curly hair into tight hair styles, which in turn causes it to break and come loose. Hair styles associated with this problem include:

- limited buns or ponytails
- braids
- cornrows
- extensions

If traction alopecia continues, a person may develop bald

places and loss of the hair.

In conditions of self-care, avoiding restricted hairstyles will most likely prevent further damage.

7. Medications

Certain medications have part results that can cause hair to fallout.

Types of such medications include:

- bloodstream thinners, such as warfarin
- Accutane, to take care of acne
- antidepressants, including Prozac and Zoloft
- beta-blockers
- cholesterol-lowering drugs, such as Lopid

If a person thinks hair loss may be due to a medication they may be taking, they should think about seeing a health care provider for an assessment. The physician could probably reduce the dose or switch the individual to another medication.

8. Nutritional deficiencies

Nutritional deficiencies can cause hair to fallout. Extreme diets that are too lower in proteins and certain nutritional vitamins, such as iron, will often cause excessive locks shedding.

A person should see a medical expert for a blood vessels test to check on if indeed they have a dietary deficiency that may be leading to their hair to fallout.

9. Birth control pills

People may experience hair loss while using contraceptive pills. Others might experience hair loss weeks or a few months once they stop taking them.

If people are taking contraceptive pills, they can pick one which has a minimal androgen index. This might help lower the chance of hair loss.

Examples of contraceptive pills with a lesser androgen index include:

- Desogen

- Ortho-Cept

- Ortho-Cyclen

- Ovral and Loestrin have an increased androgen index.

Other kinds of contraceptive that affect the hormones, such as implants and skin patches, could also cause hair loss.

The American HAIR LOSS Association recommend that individuals who have an elevated threat of genetic hair loss decide on a non-hormonal kind of birth control.

10. Ringworm

Ringworm is a fungal contamination that can cause hair loss. Ringworm on the head, or tinea capitis, can cause short-term bald areas on the top.

Symptoms include:

- a little spot that gets bigger, leading to scaly, bald

patches of skin.

- brittle hair that breaks easily.

- itchy, red patches of pores and skin in the affected areas.

- oozing blisters on the scalp.

- ring-like patches, with a red outdoors and the within of the circle coordinating your skin tone

If ringworm will not heal alone, a doctor may prescribe an antifungal medicine. On the other hand, they could prescribe an antibiotic, such as Griseofulvin.

Self-care

To prevent hair loss, people may choose to try:

- lifestyle changes to lessen stress.

- eating a nutritious diet which includes proteins, fat, and certain minerals and vitamins

The following also may help to avoid further hair loss:

- using a lightweight shampoo and conditioner to avoid weighing down the hair

- staying away from tight hairstyles.

- limiting the utilization of heating functions that may damage the hair

How do doctors classify hair loss?

You'll find so many ways to categorize hair loss. One must first examine the head to see whether the hair loss is because of the physical damage and lack of hair roots (scarring or cicatricial alopecia). If the head appears flawlessly normal with a lot of empty hair roots, this is named non-scarring hair loss. Alternatively, cicatricial alopecia completely destroys the follicles. Non-scarring hair loss also happens in situations where there is physical or chemical substance harm to the curly hair shaft, leading to breakage. Occasionally, it might be necessary to execute a biopsy of the head to tell apart these conditions. Sometimes, your physician may draw a curly hair to examine the looks of the locks shaft as well as the percentage of growing hairs (anagen stage). This article will focus on the non-scarring types of hair loss.

Patchy hair loss

Some conditions produce small regions of hair loss, while some affect large regions of the head. Common factors behind patchy hair loss are

- alopeciareata (small round or gold coin size bald areas on the head that always grow back again within several weeks),

- grip alopecia (loss from tight braids or ponytails),

- trichotillomania (the habit of twisting or pulling curly hair out),

- tinea capitis (fungal illness), and

- secondary syphilis.

Diffuse hair loss

Some common factors behind diffuse hair loss are

- pattern alopecia,

- drug-induced alopecia,

- proteins malnutrition

- systemic disease-induced alopecia (cancer, endocrine disease, and telogen effluvium).

Chapter 2

19 Herbal Treatments For Hair Regrowth

Does it certainly work?

Hair loss is a common concern for most women and men. There are multiple reasons hair may fallout, from genetics and vitamin deficiencies, to hormonal changes. Some medical ailments, such as thyroid disease, could also cause locks to slim or fallout.

There's no magic pill for growing curly hair, but research shows some herbs may decrease hair loss or help promote new development. It's important to notice however, that a lot of the study has been done on pets. Additional studies are had a need to prove their performance on humans.

Continue reading to understand how herbal treatments enable you to assist in improving your hair regrowth. Make sure to speak to your doctor before adding natural herbs to your day to day routine, particularly if your hair loss is the effect of a medical condition.

- **Natural hair oils**

Hair oils, also known as locks tonics, are natural components mixed in a carrier essential oil base. Some curly hair natural oils include multiple herbal products and carrier natural oils.

Popular carrier oils used to make organic oils are:

- coconut oil.

- nice almond oil.

- walnut oil

- olive oil.

- mineral oil.

- jojoba oil.

- whole wheat germ oil

Some herbs found in herbal hair natural oils are:

- Chinese hibiscus (Hibiscus rosa sinensis): Chinese language hibiscus can be an evergreen shrub. Its edible, lively flowers can be used to make natural tea. Hibiscus is considered to help stimulate hair roots, increase follicle size, and increase hair regrowth.

- Brahmi (Bacopa monnieri): Brahmi, also known as bacopa, is a creeping herb found in Ayurveda medicine. It includes alkaloids considered to activate protein responsible for locks growth.

- Coat buttons(Tridax procumbent):Coating control keys is a creeping Ayurvedic plant and person in the daisy family. It includes antioxidants and promotes hair regrowth alone and in synergy with other herbal remedies.

- Jatamansi (Nardostachys jatamansi):Jatamansi is a little shrub whose rhizomes may speed hair regrowth. It's been proven to increase hair regrowth in alopecia triggered by chemotherapy.

- Ginseng (Panax ginseng): Ginseng can be an age-old natural treatment for most conditions, including hair loss. It includes saponins, that are thought to encourage hair regrowth by inhibiting 5a reductase. That is an enzyme related to hair loss in men.

How exactly to use

Some hair oils are developed to use as a shampoo or a leave-in hair treatment, so observe the manufacturer's instructions. The label will help you on whether to use to moist or dry curly hair.

Using clean hands, massage therapy the hair oil right to your head and wash as directed.

- **Polyherbal ointments**

Organic ointments, sometimes called organic salves, are usually created by combining herbs with an oil like lanolin or vaseline and water. Other elements can include beeswax or cocoa butter. Polyherbal ointments typically contain multiple natural extracts.

Some herbs found in polyherbal ointments are:

- Gooseberry (Emblica officinalis): Gooseberry can be an Ayurvedic natural herb. It's used to strengthen locks and promote hair regrowth. It's also recognized to contain several antioxidants.

- Gotu kola (Centellasiatica): Gotu kola is one of the very most popular Ayurvedic natural herbs. It's considered to increase curly hair size and stimulate hair regrowth, possibly by increasing blood flow to the head.

- Aloe vera (A. Barbadensis Mill.): Aloe vera is a tropical herb and a favorite folk treatment for burns up and digestive problems. It might be also used to keep carefully the head conditioned and healthy which can support healthy hair regrowth.

- Holy basil (Ocimum sanctum): Holy basil is a fragrant, adaptogenic vitamin known because of its therapeutic properties. It could help prevent hair loss triggered by dandruff and scratching or changes in hormonal quantity.

How exactly to use

Polyherbal ointments are usually applied right to your scalp. With clean hands, therapeutic massage the ointment into the scalp until assimilated according to manufacturer's instructions.

- **Herbal creams**

Natural creams are also created from herb-infused oils and water. They contain less essential oil and more drinking water than organic ointments and are often absorbed by your skin layer.

Some herbs used to make herbal lotions are:

- Giant dodder (Cuscuta reflexa Roxb): In accordance to a 2008 studyTrusted Source, giant dodder - a sprawling, Ayurvedic flower - helps treat alopecia caused by steroid hormones by inhibiting the 5a reductase enzyme.

- Bitter apple (Citrullus colocynthis): Bitter apple is a desert, fruit-bearing vegetable found in Ayurveda. Its dried out fruit pulp is utilized to treat hair loss. Bitter apple consists of glycosides, that are compounds considered to initiate hair regrowth.

- Fake daisy (Ecliptalba): Fake daisy can be an herb found in Ayurveda to increase hair regrowth. According to a report from 2014, fake daisy helps activate hair roots and provokes a faster hair regrowth stage in nude mice.

- Night-flowering jasmine (Nyctanthes arbortristis): This small, flowering shrub is indigenous to Southern Asia. Relating to 2016 research, night-flowering jasmine initiated hair regrowth in rats and could succeed against alopecia.

How exactly to use

With clean hands, therapeutic massage the hair cream into the scalp or connect with hair from origins to tips according to manufacturer's instructions.

- **Herbal gels**

Organic gels contain natural extracts in a gel bottom. They typically don't contain essential oil.

Herbs found in organic gels to aid healthy hair can include:

- Fenugreek (Trigonella foenum-graecum): Fenugreek is an associate of the pea family. It's a favorite cooking food spice with potential hair-growing benefits. Regarding to analyze from 2006, fenugreek seed draw out improved hair quantity and hair width in women and men with moderate hair loss.

- Marking nut (Semecarpus anacardium): This herb is situated in the sub-Himalayan areand found in Ayurvedic and Siddha medication to help locks grow. More research is necessary on marking nut to determine its efficiency and safety.

How exactly to use

Using clean hands, massage therapy the gel into the scalp or connect with nice hair from root base to tips according to manufacturer's instructions.

- **Cubosomal suspension**

Cubosomes are water, crystalline nanoparticles. Cubosomal suspensions are accustomed to focus on the delivery of drugs and, in some instances, herbal remedies.

Some herbs found in cubosomal suspensions for hair regrowth are:

- Oriental arborvitae (Thuja orientalis): Oriental arborvitae can be an evergreen tree and person in the cypress family. It's a normal remedy for hair loss. Relating to a 2013 studyTrusted Source, the plant helps hair develop by stimulating the development stage in relaxing hair follicles.

- Espinosilla (Loeselia mexicana): Espinosilla is grown in Mexico. It's used to strengthen hair roots and help maintain a wholesome scalp. Regarding to a 2014 research, espinosilla demonstrated some hair regrowth in man mice.

- Goji berry (Lycium chinense Mill): This fruit-bearing shrub can be used in traditional Chinese language medicine to market hair regrowth. Goji berry includes zinc, a nutrient considered to infuse the head with essential oil to assist in preventing dandruff which can result in hair loss.

- Tuber fleeceflower (Polygonum multiflorum): This tuber is a normal Chinese medicine treatment for hair loss. It contains substances that inhibit 5a reductase enzymes. In addition, it helps promote the development stage in hair roots.

How exactly to use

Using clean hands, comb in or connect with hair from underlying to hint, or as otherwise instructed. Use natural cubosomal suspensions as aimed by your physician.

Possible side effects and risks

The main threat of herbal hair regrowth products is allergic attack. You should execute a patch test to check on for an allergic attack before using any herbal products.

To get this done:

1. Apply a little amount of product to the within of your wrist.

2. Leave on for at least a day.

3. In the event that you haven't experienced any irritation within per day, it ought to be safe to use elsewhere.

In the event that you do develop an allergic attack, you might experience:

- Rash.

- Hives.

- Redness.

- Itching.

- difficulty breathing.

- Dizziness.

- headache

Potential side effect of topical organic hair regrowth products include:

- Thinning hair

- increased hair loss

- dry scalp

- scalp inflammation or irritation

The side effect of most herbs for hair regrowth aren't well-studied in humans. There's insufficient information to standardize dosing suggestions.

Women who are pregnant or breastfeeding shouldn't use herbal remedies to grow curly hair unless under the guidance of a health care provider or a professional natural physician.

The bottom line

No herbal treatment can regrow a complete tresses. You

ought to be wary of natural products that state to be always a hair growth feeling.

Research shows that some natural herbs can help strengthen locks, support head health, improve curly hair width, or stimulate the hair regrowth routine. Still, more medical tests on humans are needed before herbal treatments become a popular hair regrowth treatment.

Any herb can be utilized in every types of herbal hair product preparations. But it could be difficult to acquire over-the-counter hair regrowth products that are the herbs found in research. Your physician or natural physician might be able to support you in finding a treatment that best suits your preferences.

Make sure to talk to your physician before use. They are able to walk you through your treatment plans and help you on any next steps.

Chapter 3

30 Natural Herbs For Hair Regrowth And Thickness

Hair loss is an universal problem that is faced by men and women, where their hair gets sparse from balding, loss hair, or a receding hairline. It manifests gradually and sometimes you don't even respect it as a problem until you've lost quite a little of hair.

Finding that you're dropping nice hair can make you stress, stress, and confusion in regards to what you must do. With so many products on the market that guarantee hair regrowth, it can often be hard to produce a choice.

Even though many products promise the goodness of herbs, it is impossible to learn the consequences of something on your scalp, considering all the chemicals that get into which makes it. So why not only consider the herbs?

The usage of herbs to take care of hair loss and promote hair regrowth has been common practice for years and years before commercial products was even considered. While commercial products guarantee the goodness of an all natural ingredient, they come packed with chemicals. This makes the utilization of herbal products a preferred solution.

There are various herbs used for hair regrowth, and each has unique properties that produce them ideal ingredients relating to hair care regime.

1) Amla or Indian Gooseberry

Scientific Name: Phyllanthus Emblica

Amla, also called the Indian Gooseberry, is a fruits

loaded with vitamin C and many other antioxidants that assist with collagen creation. Collagen improves the rate of which locks develops and ensures strong hair regrowth. Dry Amla natural powder can be blended with coconut essential oil and put on your hair. You can even combine the natural powder with water to create a paste. The paste can be employed to nice hair as a locks mask. Allow it sit down for at least thirty minutes and then wash it off with cold water.

Benefit Of Amla:

- Promotes hair regrowth

- Reduces hair graying

- Supports dandruff and head condition

- Acts as curly hair conditioner

2) Shikakai

Scientific Name: Acacia Concinna

Shikakai comes from the bark, leaves, and pods of the Shikakai tree. Its natural powder helps to improve locks, control dandruff and softly cleanse the head. It's mostly found in the same manner as Amla. It could be found in its powdered form with a carrier essential oil like coconut, or it could be used as a curly hair mask by combining the powdered Shikakai in drinking water to create a paste. Dried out Shikakai fruits is also steeped in drinking water to get ready a healing facial cleanser. That is one of the very most effective herbal remedies that promote hair regrowth.

Benefit Of Shikakai

- Cleanses and enhances the fitness of your scalp
- Controls Dandruff
- Promotes hair regrowth
- Strengthens roots of hairs

3) Reetha or Cleaning soap Nuts

Scientific Name: Sapindus

Reetha tops the set of natural herbs that promote hair regrowth. Reetha, also called cleaning soap nut products, are fruits that are dried out and used entire or in natural powder form. The fruits of the Reetha tree have been used to make soaps for a long period, and that's where their name, cleaning soap nuts was produced from. Reetha is soaked in boiling drinking water, and the producing liquid is utilized to clean curly hair. It really is an effective remedy for hair loss.

Benefit Of Reetha:

- Nourishes the hair roots and scalp
- Promotes healthy hair regrowth
- Cleanses the scalp
- Anti-inflammatory properties battle away infections.

4) Henna

Scientific Name: Lawsonia inermis

Henna is often for hair color, but it addittionally works like a charm for the entire health of hair. They have antibacterial, antimicrobial, and astringent properties. It gets rid of excess natural oils from the head, avoiding clogging. Henna leaves are powdered, blended with drinking water, and rested for a couple of hours. The paste is then put on the locks and left set for a few hours. It really is rinsed off with drinking water.

Benefit Of Henna:

- Natural hair dye
- Treats greasy hair
- Restores the pH degree of the scalp
- Repairs damage

5) Methi or Fenugreek

Scientific Name: Trigonella foenum-graecum

Methi or fenugreek is nature's conditioner. The seed products are soaked in drinking water; the resulting water is a slimy material that is put into an assortment of Shikakai, Amla, and henna. Additionally, the seed products can be soaked in drinking water over night and then floor to an excellent paste and put on the hair. You can include just a little yogurt to the paste, to reap the advantages of the added lactic acidity.

Benefit Of Methi:

- Improves blood circulation in the scalp
- Promotes hair regrowth
- Conditions the hair

6) Brahmi

Scientific Name: Bacopa Monnieri

Brahmi can be used in essential oil and natural powder form to avoid hair loss and make curly hair thicker and healthier. The natural powder is blended with water to create a paste and it is put on the locks and head for one hour. A mind therapeutic massage with Brahmi essential oil is the perfect stress-buster that reduces hair loss.

Benefit Of Brahmi:

- Reduces stress and hair loss
- Promotes hair regrowth

- Nourishes the scalp

7) Neem

Scientific Name: Azadirachta indica

Neem oil improves the rate of hair regrowth and escalates the tensile strength of the curly hair shafts, making them silky and adding sparkle. It reduces hair loss and discomfort of the head (4). Neem leaf pastes can be utilized as conditioning packages to nourish the head and stop dryness and flaking.

Benefit Of Neem:

- Controls Dandruff

- Cleanses and nourishes the scalp

- Antibacterial properties keep infections away

8) Horsetail

Scientific Name: Equisetum arvense

Horsetail is a highly effective component for promoting hair regrowth and maintaining the fitness of your head. It stimulates arteries and improves blood flow (5). Steeping two parts drinking water with one part dried out horsetail, will provide you with a remedy that you can connect with your hair.

Benefit of Horsetail:

- Improves flow by stimulating arteries
- Increases tensile power of hair loss

9) Bhringraj

Scientific Name: Eclipta Alba

This is a historical Ayurvedic remedy that is in use for years and years in India. It is utilized to treat hair loss and also to rejuvenate the head. You should use this natural herb with the addition of Bhringraj natural powder to a carrier essential oil and then applying the combination to nice hair. When you have fresh Bhringraj leaves, grind them and apply the paste straight onto your locks.

Benefit Bhringraj:

- Promotes new hair regrowth.

- Adds glow and luster to hair

10) Lavender

Scientific Name: Lavendula officinalis

Lavender is well known because of its distinctive but enjoyable aroma. It can be used in curly hair look after its anti-inflammatory and anti-microbial properties. It really is an all natural insect repellent that protects the locks from lice. You should use lavender gas with the addition of a few drops to a carrier essential oil of your decision.

Benefit of Lavender:

- Controls essential oil production
- Natural insect repellant
- Keeps the head healthy

11) Flaxseed

Scientific Name: Linum usitatissimum

Flaxseed contains a good amount of essential fatty acids which are crucial for hair. In addition, it includes antioxidants that be rid of free radicals. To use flaxseed for nice hair, boil surface seeds to create a gel. Apply this gel to your head and hair.

Benefit of Flaxseed:

- Nourishes hair

- Battles free radicals

- Strengthens hair

- Prevents hair loss

- Moisturizes hair

12) Nettle

Scientific Name: Urtica dioica

Nettle is a highly effective solution to treatment hair loss since it stimulates the head and improves blood flow. In addition, it strengthens the curly hair shafts. Nettle can be floor to produce a paste. Blend this paste with essential olive oil and use it to hair.

Benefit of Nettle:

- Prevents hair loss

- Improves circulation

- Reduces harm and breakage

13) Found Palmetto

Scientific Name: Serenoa repens

Saw Palmetto halts the testosterone from being changed into dihydrotestosterone. Dihydrotestosterone may be associated with hair loss (8). The vitamin, therefore, prevents hair loss and stimulates healthy hair regrowth. Noticed Palmetto can be studied by means of vitamins. You can even rinse nice hair with this plant.

Benefits Of saw Palmetto:

- Reduces hair loss

- Nourishes locks and scalp

14) Calendula

Scientific Name: Calendula officincilis

Calendula is additionally known as Marigold and can be an abundant way to obtain vitamins, nutrients, and antioxidants that help combat inflammation. It improves the creation of collagen which boosts blood flow in the head and promotes healthy hair regrowth. It does increase the tensile power of the curly hair shaft and can be utilized only or with a moisturizing carrier essential oil.

Benefit of Calendula:

- Nourishes locks and scalp
- Increases collagen
- Improves blood flow

15) Comfrey

Scientific Name: Symphytum officinale

Comfrey is among the best herbs for hair regrowth and its draw out is utilized for detangling curly hair. It contains minerals and vitamins that help out with healthy hair regrowth. Comfrey stimulates and soothes the head. It protects against dryness and breaking. You should use comfrey as a locks wash by boiling one teaspoon of dried out comfrey in a single glass of boiling drinking water. Add one tablespoon of apple cider vinegar to the perfect solution is. After the solution has cooled, put it over newly washed hair.

Benefit of Comfrey:

- Promotes healthy hair regrowth.

- Stimulates the scalp

- Reduces Dryness

- Detangles hair

16) Chamomile

Scientific Name: Matricaria recutitia

Chamomile is well known because of its soothing aroma, though it is often consumed as tea, it may also be used externally for locks care. It really is recognized to nourish and soothe the head, encouraging healthy hair regrowth. Additionally it is an all natural highlighter that can truly add light shades to hair. You should use chamomile by rinsing nice hair with the teafter it's been newly cleaned and conditioned.

Benefit of Chamomile:

- Soothes the scalp
- Nourishes the roots

17) Arnica

Scientific Name: Arnica montana

The anti-inflammatory properties in Arnica make it a good herb to keep up the fitness of your scalp (9). It really is a great ingredient to use to fight dandruff. A wholesome head leads to healthy hair regrowth. Arnica essential oil can be employed right to the head or in mixture with some other carrier oil.

Benefit of Arnica:

- Anti-inflammatory

- Controls dandruff
- Promotes hair regrowth

18) Gotu Kola

Scientific Name: Centellasiatica

Gotu kola blended with olive oil is great for head massages. It does increase blood flow and hair regrowth. The increased blood flow nourishes the head which boosts hair regrowth and curbs hair loss.

Benefit of Gotu Kola:

- Improves blood flow
- Promotes curly hair re-growth

19) Dandelion

Scientific Name: Taraxacum officinale

The dandelion herb is abundant with iron and Vitamin A, both which are crucial for treating conditions of the scalp. Ensuring head health is paramount to promoting hair regrowth. Dandelion tea, created by boiling one tablespoon of dandelion in 2 mugs of drinking water for ten minutes, can be utilized as a curly hair rinse.

Benefit of Dandelion:

- Controls Dandruff
- Promotes hair regrowth

20) Licorice

Scientific Name: Glycyrrhiza glabra

Licorice main has triterpene saponins, glycosides, and flavonoids, that nourish the head and heal any harm that may have been caused by fungal disease. It works as a highly effective facial cleanser. To use licorice main as a locks cleanser, add one tablespoon from it to three mugs of boiling drinking water. Allow it simmer for one hour and then stress it. After it cools, apply the answer to your head and hair.

Benefit of Licorice:

- Nourish the scalp

- Heal damage

21) Yucca

Scientific Name: Yucca schidigera

Yucca is a plant that is local to the UNITED STATES deserts. It really is typically used as an all natural head cleanser and it is also used to make soaps and hair shampoo as it effectively fights scratching, dryness, and dandruff. Yucca can be blended with drinking water to make a highly effective hair rinse.

Benefit of Yucca:

- Cleanses the scalp
- Prevents dryness

22) Hops

Scientific Name: Humulus lupulus

Hops is a well-known hair regrowth stimulant. It is utilized in essential oil form to thicken locks and promote hair regrowth. Additionally it is an all natural antiseptic.

To use hops, blend it with a carrier essential oil of your decision and use it to hair.

Benefit of Hops:

- Thickens hair

- Improves Blood flow

- Natural antiseptic

23) Peppermint

Scientific Name: Mentha piperita

Peppermint can be an antifungal and anti-inflammatory natural herb that is well known because of its moisturizing properties. It really is commonly found in the proper execution of essential oil, which is put on the head and hair and it is a known hair regrowth booster. It improves the blood circulation, increasing the nourishment the follicles get. To include peppermint to nice hair care and attention routine, combine a few drops from it to a carrier essential oil and use it to your head and hair.

Benefit of Peppermint:

- Antifungal
- Anti-inflammatory
- Improves blood flow
- Combats itchiness and inflammation

24) Cassia

Scientific Name: Cassia obovata

Cassia is a well-known conditioner for dry out hair. It really is sometimes known as the blonde henna since it provides fantastic hues to grey curly hair. To use cassia, blend cassia in drinking water until it reaches a pasty regularity. Apply the paste to hair and allow it sit down for one hour. Wash nice hair to eliminate any residue.

Benefit of Cassia:

- Antibacterial
- Reduces hair loss

- Conditions hair

25) Marshmallow

Scientific Name: Althaea officinalis

The roots of marshmallow contain lauric acid and essential fatty acids that can be found in coconut oil, rendering it a great ingredient that nourishes the hair and promotes hair regrowth. To use marshmallow main, boil marshmallow in drinking water for quarter-hour. Strain the water and add it to your conditioner for use.

Benefit of Marshmallow:

- Nourishes hair

- Promotes healthy hair regrowth

- Detangles hair

26) Thyme

Scientific Name: Thymus vulgaris

Thyme is a herb that is abundant with potassium, magnesium, and selenium. It can help induce the follicles which lead to hair re-growth. They have antiseptic and anti-fungal properties that assist maintain head health. Thyme essential oil can be blended with a carrier essential oil and applied. You can even rinse hair with thyme by steeping it in drinking water, straining it, and then allowing it to cool.

Benefit of Thyme:

- Promotes hair regrowth

- Antiseptic

- Antifungal

27) Parsley

Scientific Name: Petroselinium crispum

Parsley improves the creation of keratin and collagen in the head, both which are crucial for hair regrowth. It increases the blood circulation and includes nutritional vitamins and antioxidants that fight damage leading to free-radicals. In addition, it helps synthesize melanin, which is the pigment that protects locks from sun-damage. Parsley can be utilized as an organic wash by boiling it in drinking water. You can even make a parsley curly hair mask by milling it into a paste with drinking water.

A word of Caution: Women that are pregnant should avoid ingesting large quantity of parsley.

Benefit of Parsley:

- Improves blood flow

- Promotes locks re-growth

- Protects from sunlight damage

28) Watercress

Scientific Name: Nasturtium officinale

Watercress has a higher content of biotin and potassium rendering it an effective hair loss treatment. It promotes active hair regrowth. In addition, it has high quantity of Vitamin A which nourish the curly hair shaft and promotes the development of new locks. To produce a watercress wash, blend a small number of watercress in a single cup of drinking water. Boil the blend for a few momemts, stress it, and allow it cool. Utilize the water as a wash on freshly cleaned hair.

Benefit of Watercress:

- Reduces hair loss
- Increases curly hair strength
- Nourishes scalp

29) Moringa

Scientific Name: Moringa oleifera

Moringa contains thiocyanate which strengthens the follicles and prevents hair loss. It can be used as a conditioner and promotes new hair regrowth. You should use moringa in its essential oil form through the use of it right to nice hair. Alternatively, you may make a tea out of moringa natural powder and utilize this to wash hair.

Benefit of Moringa:

- Reduces HAIR LOSS
- Promotes hair growth

30) Maidenhair

Scientific Name: Ginko Biloba

Maidenhair, as the name suggests, is a favorite locks care herb. It really is a highly effective treatment for hair loss as it enhances the blood circulation to the head. To create an infusion of maidenhair which you can use to wash nice hair, add three handfuls of the dried out vitamin to 2 mugs of drinking water and allow it boil. Stress the water and carefully put it over newly washed hair.

Benefit of Maidenhair:

- Increases blood flow
- Promotes new hair growth
- Adds shine

16 Wonder Herbs That Prevent Hair Loss

Hair loss-the two words that are dreaded by women and men alike. There are many factors that can cause hair loss in women, which range from psychological or physical stress, starting a fresh medication, bad curly hair health, auto-immune diseases, dietary deficiencies, fever or disease, etc. Sometimes it could be multiple factors working collectively that cause hair to fallout. It's usually difficult to pinpoint the precise cause unless you're identified as having an auto-immune disease or are on medication that's recognized to cause hair loss as a side-effect.

Aside from maintaining a healthy diet plan and showing nice hair some much-needed TLC, there are many ways to counter-top hair loss and restore hair to the former glory. One particular method incorporates the utilization of Ayurvedic herbal products that have always been used to deal with hair fall. Pursuing is a summary of 16 herbal remedies and ways to use them to take care of hair loss.

16 Best Herbs For Hair Loss Treatment

1. Aloe Vera

You'll need

- 2 tbsp Aloe Vera Gel

Processing Time

- 2 hours

Process

- Cut the Aloe Vera stem and scoop out 2 tablespoons of gel.

- Apply the extracted gel to your head and lightly massage it for two minutes.

- Leave the gel in nice hair for 2 hours and then clean it off using a mild shampoo.

How Often?

- Continue doing this twice weekly.

Why This Works

Aloe Vera restores head health by fitness it while balancing sebum creation and pH quantity. This, not only curbs hair loss, but it addittionally promotes locks re-growth.

2. Ginseng

You'll need

- 2-3 tbsp Ginseng Infused Oil

Processing Time

- 45 minutes

Process

- Pour three tablespoons of the Ginseng infused essential oil into a dish.

- Section hair and begin massaging the oil into the scalp.

- Work the essential oil into your curly hair until the entire amount of it is protected.

- Massage your head for ten minutes.

- Leave the oil in nice hair for yet another thirty minutes and then wash it out with a mild shampoo.

How Often?

- Continue doing this thrice weekly.

Why This Works

Ginseng is thought to stimulate blood flow, thus increasing the way to obtain blood and nourishment to the hair roots. This enables for healthy hair regrowth.

3. Rosemary

You'll need

- 5-10 drops Rosemary GAS
- 2-3 tbsp Carrier Oil

Processing Time

- 45 minutes

Process

- In a dish, combine the rosemary gas with a carrier oil (such as coconut, olive, almond, or jojoba) of your decision.

- Massage this essential oil blend into the head and work it through your locks.

- Massage your head for ten minutes

- Leave the oil in hair for yet another thirty minutes and then wash it out with a mild shampoo.

How Often?

- Continue doing this thrice weekly.

Why This Works

Rosemary is a robust herb for hair regrowth. It not only prevents hair loss but also stimulates new hair regrowth, detoxifies head and restores curly hair pigment.

4. Indian Gooseberry

You'll need

- 4 tbsp Indian Gooseberry Powder
- 2 tsp Lemon Juice
- Water

Processing Time

- 20 minutes

Process

- In a dish, add water to the Indian Gooseberry natural powder and lemon juice until you get a clean, consistent paste.
- Massage this into the scalp and use it to the complete amount of your hair.
- Let it sit down for quarter-hour and wash it out with a mild shampoo.

How Often?

- Continue doing this twice weekly.

Why This Works

Indian gooseberry, also called "Amla," is abundant with Vitamin C and other nutrients such as phosphorus, calcium mineral, iron, Vitamin B complicated and carotene. It promotes hair regrowth, strengthens roots of hairs, and increases sparkle.

Amla juice, when blended with drinking water, helps restore the vitality of locks, while offering power and sparkle. Gooseberry can control dandruff, prevents extreme hair loss and early graying. The addition of some Amla natural powder to Henna combine offers conditioning and restorative properties.

5. Neem

You'll need

- A couple of Neem Leaves

- 2 cups Water

Processing Time

- 5 minutes

Process

- Boil the neem leaves in 2 mugs of drinking water for ten minutes. Set this apart to cool.

- After the solution has cooled off, strain the water into a jug.

- Wash nice hair with a mild shampoo and then put the neem infused drinking water through it as your final rinse.

- Do not wash hair further.

How Often?

- Do this after every wash.

Why This Works

Neem has high anti-bacterial properties which are of help as it pertains to remedying an itchy, dandruff-prone head. It improves blood flow to the head when applied topically. Neem essential oil is effective in tackling hair loss and early graying. In addition, it boosts hair regrowth, and prevents and remedies many curly hair problems.

Dry Neem natural powder can be blended with water to produce a solid paste, which is massaged in to the head to exfoliate, cleanse and nourish the head. Nearly thirty minutes before shampooing will offer you benefits. Remember that the primary of Neem essential oil is strong, and therefore, it ought to be blended with a lighter essential oil such as olive, coconut, and almond before software.

6. Sage

You'll need

- 2 tbsp Dried Sage Leaves

- 2 cups Water

Processing Time

- 5 mins

Process

- Boil the dried sage leaves in 2 mugs of drinking water for ten minutes. Set this apart to cool.

- After the solution has cooled off, strain the water into a jug.

- Wash nice hair with a mild shampoo and then put the sage infused drinking water through it as your final rinse.

- Do not wash hair further.

How Often?

- Do this after each wash.

Why This Works

Sage has antiseptic and astringent benefits for the locks. Regular use of the plant results in heavier and stronger curly hair.

7. Burdock

You'll need

- 2 drops Rosemary GAS
- 2 drops Basil GAS
- 2 drops Lavender GAS
- 1 tsp Aloe Vera Gel
- 1 tsp Burdock Oil

Processing Time

- 2 hours

Process

- Combine all the substances in a dish.

- Start rubbing the essential oil blend into the scalp.

- Massage your head for a few momemts and then leave the essential oil mixture set for a few hours.

- Wash it out with a mild hair shampoo.

How Often?

- Continue doing this thrice weekly.

Why This Works

Burdock root essential oil extract is abundant with phytosterols and efa's, the nutrition that must maintain a wholesome head and promote natural hair regrowth.

8. Bhringraj

You'll need

- A couple of Bhringraj Leaves

- 1 cup Coconut/Sesame Oil

Processing Time

- 45 minutes

Process

- Finely chop the bhringraj leaves and heat them in a saucepan with the oil.

- Keep the essential oil on heating for ten minutes and then arranged it apart to cool.

- After the oil is cool, section nice hair and begin massaging the oil into the scalp.

- Work the right path down with the essential oil before whole amount of hair is covered.

- Wait for thirty minutes and then wash the essential oil out with hair shampoo.

- Store the surplus essential oil away for later use.

How Often?

- Continue doing this thrice weekly.

Why This Works

Bhringaraj is one of the very most powerful herbs used to treatment hair loss and premature graying. It leads to healthy hair, a wholesome head and promotes locks re-growth.

9. Jatamansi

You'll need

- 5 drops Jatamansi GAS
- 2 tbsp Carrier Essential oil (Coconut/Sesame)

Processing Time

- 45 minutes

Process

- Combine the natural oils in a dish to make a Jatamansi oil mix.

- Start massaging this essential oil into your head and work the right path right down to the tips of hair.

- Massage your head for yet another 10 minutes.

- Wait around, with the essential oil in nice hair, for around 30 minutes at least and then wash it out with hair shampoo.

How Often?

- Continue doing this thrice weekly.

Why This Works

Jatamansi infused with essential oil is very useful as it pertains to preventing hair loss and premature graying due to its bloodstream purifying properties.

10. Curry Leaves

You'll need

- A small number of Curry Leaves

- 2 tbsp Coconut Oil

Processing Time

- 45 minutes

Process

- Heat the oil and curry leaves in a saucepan before oil starts to defend myself against a brown color.

- Allow curry leaves infused essential oil cool and then start massaging it into the scalp and use it to the space of hair.

- Leave this essential oil set for at least thirty minutes. You can even leave it in right away.

- Rinse the essential oil out with hair shampoo.

How Often?

- Continue doing this thrice weekly.

Why This Works

Curry leaves are generally used to avoid premature

graying, stimulate hair regrowth and nourish the root base.

11. Holy Basil

You'll need

- A small number of holy basil leaves
- 2-3 tbsp essential olive oil

Processing Time

- 45 minutes

Process

- Dry out the basil leaves in sunlight and then check out grind these to a fine natural powder.
- Blend the basil natural powder with somewhat preheated essential olive oil.
- Sieve the oil in a muslin cloth and then start applying the oil to your head and hair.

- Massage your head for ten minutes and leave the essential oil in for yet another 30 minutes.

- Rinse the essential oil out with hair shampoo.

- If you make large quantity of this essential oil, you can store it in a jar or container with a good cap and stick it in the refrigerator. The essential oil can be stored for 11 times.

How Often?

- Continue doing this thrice weekly.

Why This Works

Holy Basil or Tulsi, as it is often known, helps rejuvenate the hair roots. Massaging Basil essential oil into the head not only moisturizes the curly hair, but it addittionally helps stimulate blood flow, that leads to improved hair regrowth. Basil is thought to contain Eugenol and magnesium, which jointly improve the blood circulation to the head.

12. Reetha (Soapnuts)

You'll need

- 6-7 Soapnuts
- 2 Indian Gooseberries
- 2 cups Water

Processing Time

- 15 minutes

Process

- Soak the soapnuts and gooseberries in 2 mugs of drinking water and leave it overnight.

- Each day, heat water with the soapnuts and gooseberries still in it until it begins to boil.

- Let the drinking water cool and then mash the soapnuts and gooseberries.

- Strain the water and utilize it to wash nice hair rather than using shampoo.

- This mixture will not lather as well as shampoo, so rather than massaging your scalp and hair, pour the Reetha water through your hair and await 5-10 minutes then check out rinse it out with water.

How Often?

Replace the hair shampoo in two of your regular washes with this natural cleanser.

Why This Works

Cleaning soap nuts or Reetha is thought to contain Saponin, an all natural cleanser which boosts scalp health insurance and restores pH quantity. This treatment helps maintains your head clean and healthy without needing severe, damage-causing chemicals.

13. Hibiscus Flower

You'll need

- 2 Hibiscus flowers

- 2 tbsp Carrier Oil

Processing Time

- 45 minutes

Process

- Warmth any oil that you utilize on hair with the hibiscus blossom for two minutes.

- Start applying this hibiscus infused essential oil onto your head and hair.

- Massage your head for ten minutes and leave the essential oil in for yet another 30 minutes.

- Clean off with shampoo.

How Often?

- Continue doing this twice weekly.

Why This Works

Hibiscus flower, aside from preventing hair loss, may add glow to the boring hair although it also battles graying of hair.

14. Ginger

You'll need

- 1 Grated Ginger Root
- 4 tbsp Sesame Oil

Processing Time

- 45 minutes

Process

- Place the grated ginger main in the muslin fabric and press or remove juice.
- Combine 1 tsp of the juice with the sesame essential oil to make a ginger oil mix.
- Massage this mix into your head and await thirty minutes before rinsing it out with a mild hair shampoo.

How Often?

- Continue doing this thrice weekly.

Why This Works

Ginger essential oil helps treat and stop dandruff. Additionally it is known to activate hair regrowth while boosting blood circulation.

15. Lemongrass

YOU'LL NEED

- 3 tsp Dried out Lemongrass
- 1 cup Water

Processing Time

5 minutes

Process

- Boil the dried lemongrass in 1 glass of drinking water and then allow it cool.

- After the solution is cool, strain the water and collection it aside.

- Clean and condition nice hair and then check out pour the lemongrass drinking water through your locks as your final rinse.

How Often?

- Continue doing this twice weekly.

Why This Works

Lemongrass strengthens the hair roots which is vital for preventing hair loss.

16. Noticed Palmetto

You'll need

- 10 drops noticed palmetto gas

- 2 tbsp essential olive oil

Processing Time

- 45 minutes

Process

1. In a dish, dilute the Noticed Palmetto oil with essential olive oil.

2. Start rubbing this essential oil blend into the scalp and use it to hair.

3. Massage nice hair for ten minutes and then wait around with the essential oil in hair for thirty minutes.

4. Wash the essential oil out of nice hair with a mild shampoo.

5. Optionally, you can eat the saw palmetto fruit to limit your hair loss problem.

How Often?

You should use this Saw Palmetto oil mix 3-4 times weekly.

Why This Works

Noticed Palmetto blocks the creation of dihydrotestosterone which really is a chemical associated with hair loss. By obstructing the creation of DHT, Noticed Palmetto motivates unhindered hair regrowth.

12 Wonderful Vegetables For Hair Regrowth

Vegetables are our close friends when we want to lose some pounds, right? What with the dieting and everything! These humbles vegetables are also ideal for our curly hair. These fruits & vegetables for hair regrowth contain nutritional vitamins, fibres and nutrients which are recognized to help with hair regrowth and keeping the consistency and smoothness.

Here I'll list down some pointers to keep the hair healthy and happy. Before that, like always, below are a few what to know before you begin with the tips

- Clean, wet hair absorbs nutritional vitamins better

than dried out, dirty hair. It could appear to be a cumbersome job to wash hair, placed on a pack and then clean it again, but its totally worthwhile. There's a reason salons offer you a hair clean before and treatment and styling.

- Using warm water starts up nice hair and head pores while cool water closes them. So use hot water before program and cool water post app.

- Avoid using warm water on hair as it drains hair of its oils and lessens the elasticity.

- Some vegetables leave a strange smell, so follow-up with your preferred conditioner to face mask the smell.

- Any cover up needs ample time for you to penetrate into the locks. Leave on the mask for atleast thirty minutes to see results.

- Also, do not over leave it. When the face mask starts drying, it could draw drinking water from curly hair and counter take action the results.

Vegetables for hair regrowth:

Now let's see a few of the most beneficial vegetables that may be included to your set of best methods for hair growth.

1. Spinach

Amongst those vegetables that are believed nutritious for nice hair, spinach tops the list. Filled with edible dietary fiber, spinach is a wealthy way to obtain iron and zinc in addition to other essential minerals and vitamins. Both of these particular nutrients are highly essential for the locks, as the lack of zinc and iron often leads to hair loss in many people.

2. Carrots:

Carrots will be the second best veggie for hair regrowth. Carrots are a wealthy store of Vitamin B7 or Biotin that is known as a wholesome tonic for the curly hair. Biotin is vital for locks re-growth. At exactly the same time, it can help to fortify the roots of hairs so that curly hair does not fallout easily.

Boil some carrots and mix them. Don't toss the drinking water you boiled them in, use the same to grind and mix them. Apply the paste to hair and leave on for thirty minutes. Clean it away. This cover up helps reduce hair loss and also promotes hair regrowth.

3. Onions:

Onions are also a helpful nutrient for the locks. It really is an affluent way to obtain zinc, iron and Biotin, which are needful for hair regrowth. Furthermore to hair regrowth, onion is an excellent veggie that helps in stopping the early graying of curly hair.

4. Sweet Potatoes:

Nice potatoes are a great way to obtain beta-carotene. The body transforms beta-carotene into Vitamin A. Beta-carotene is necessary for cellular repair in the body. Nice potatoes match the dearth of Vitamin A to a big extent.

5. **Tomatoes:**

Tomatoes are high resources of antioxidants. Antioxidants are also effective cell-repairing brokers. They help remove harmful particles and harmful toxins from the top of scalp. You can either consume tomato vegetables straight or apply the tomato pulp on the head for greater results. Tomatoes help improve the stand out and luster of the locks.

6. **Garlic:**

Although using a pungent smell, garlic is a perfect tonic for the hair. It really is good to include this to your regular diet graph, as it includes very few calorie consumption. In addition, garlic clove contains an extremely high sulfur content, which is known as best for curly hair re-growth.

7. Beetroots:

Using a red-colored veggie raises your lycopene, which may increase hair regrowth rate. Beetroots contain lycopene that really helps to stimulate hair regrowth. Furthermore to beetroots, the majority of the reddish vegetables are best for the locks, as they could support the same nutrient.

8. Curry Leaves:

Relatively less discussed, curry leaves are a great antidote for hair loss. Curry leaves contain keratin, which is known as a perfect tonic for hair regrowth and will be offering you lustrous curly hair.

9. French Coffee beans:

French beans will be the richest way to obtain Vitamins A and E. Vitamin Electronic is highly needful for enhancing the luster and level of hair. In addition, it protects nice hair from premature graying.

10. Green Chili:

Another wealthy store of keratin and Vitamin E, green chilies are great for fostering hair regrowth. It also really helps to repair the broken cellular material of the head in order to market new hair roots.

11. Orange veggie offer you beta substances which also help achieve healthy long locks. They reduce curly hair breakage and hair loss. Get your dosage of beta carotene from oranges and yellow coloured vegetables - bell peppers is a superb source.

12. Cucumber is also recognized to achieve healthy locks. Merge some fresh cucumbers and apply the paste to your head and massage completely. You might like to then add fenugreek natural powder as mix will be runny.

Acknowledgements

The Glory of this book success goes to God Almighty and my beautiful Family, Fans, Readers & well-wishers, Customers, and Friends for their endless support and encouragement.

www.ingramcontent.com/pod-product-compliance
Lightning Source LLC
Chambersburg PA
CBHW020301030426
42336CB00010B/859